THIS BOOK BELONGS TO

CURRENT WEIGHT

TARGET WEIGHT

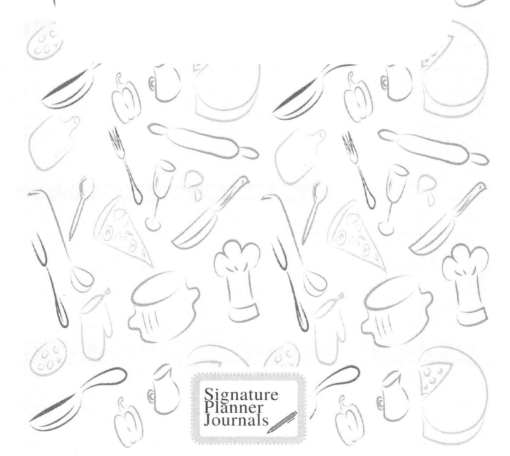

Signature
Planner
Journals

DATE	MONDAY
B'Fast	
Lunch	
Dinner	
Snacks	

DATE	TUESDAY
B'Fast	
Lunch	
Dinner	
Snacks	

DATE	WEDNESDAY
B'Fast	
Lunch	
Dinner	
Snacks	

DATE	THURSDAY
B'Fast	
Lunch	
Dinner	
Snacks	

WEEK	DATE	WEIGHT	+/-

HEALTH GOALS

	FRIDAY	DATE
B'Fast		
Lunch		
Dinner		
Snacks		

	SATURDAY	DATE
B'Fast		
Lunch		
Dinner		
Snacks		

	SUNDAY	DATE
B'Fast		
Lunch		
Dinner		
Snacks		

WATER TRACKER

M	○	○	○	○	○	○	○
T	○	○	○	○	○	○	○
W	○	○	○	○	○	○	○
T	○	○	○	○	○	○	○
F	○	○	○	○	○	○	○
S a	○	○	○	○	○	○	○
S u	○	○	○	○	○	○	○

SHOPPING LIST

-
-
-
-
-
-
-
-
-
-

DATE	MONDAY
B'Fast	
Lunch	
Dinner	
Snacks	

DATE	TUESDAY
B'Fast	
Lunch	
Dinner	
Snacks	

DATE	WEDNESDAY
B'Fast	
Lunch	
Dinner	
Snacks	

DATE	THURSDAY
B'Fast	
Lunch	
Dinner	
Snacks	

WEEK	DATE	WEIGHT	+/-

HEALTH GOALS

FRIDAY	DATE
B'Fast	
Lunch	
Dinner	
Snacks	

SATURDAY	DATE
B'Fast	
Lunch	
Dinner	
Snacks	

SUNDAY	DATE
B'Fast	
Lunch	
Dinner	
Snacks	

WATER TRACKER

M	○	○	○	○	○	○	○
T	○	○	○	○	○	○	○
W	○	○	○	○	○	○	○
T	○	○	○	○	○	○	○
F	○	○	○	○	○	○	○
Sa	○	○	○	○	○	○	○
Su	○	○	○	○	○	○	○

SHOPPING LIST

-
-
-
-
-
-
-
-
-

DATE	MONDAY
B'Fast	
Lunch	
Dinner	
Snacks	

DATE	TUESDAY
B'Fast	
Lunch	
Dinner	
Snacks	

DATE	WEDNESDAY
B'Fast	
Lunch	
Dinner	
Snacks	

DATE	THURSDAY
B'Fast	
Lunch	
Dinner	
Snacks	

WEEK	DATE	WEIGHT	+/-

HEALTH GOALS

FRIDAY		DATE
B'Fast		
Lunch		
Dinner		
Snacks		

SATURDAY		DATE
B'Fast		
Lunch		
Dinner		
Snacks		

SUNDAY		DATE
B'Fast		
Lunch		
Dinner		
Snacks		

WATER TRACKER

M	○	○	○	○	○	○	○
T	○	○	○	○	○	○	○
W	○	○	○	○	○	○	○
T	○	○	○	○	○	○	○
F	○	○	○	○	○	○	○
Sa	○	○	○	○	○	○	○
Su	○	○	○	○	○	○	○

SHOPPING LIST

-
-
-
-
-
-
-
-
-
-

DATE	MONDAY
B'Fast	
Lunch	
Dinner	
Snacks	

DATE	TUESDAY
B'Fast	
Lunch	
Dinner	
Snacks	

DATE	WEDNESDAY
B'Fast	
Lunch	
Dinner	
Snacks	

DATE	THURSDAY
B'Fast	
Lunch	
Dinner	
Snacks	

WEEK	DATE	WEIGHT	+/-

HEALTH GOALS

	FRIDAY	DATE
B'Fast		
Lunch		
Dinner		
Snacks		

	SATURDAY	DATE
B'Fast		
Lunch		
Dinner		
Snacks		

	SUNDAY	DATE
B'Fast		
Lunch		
Dinner		
Snacks		

WATER TRACKER

M	○	○	○	○	○	○	○
T	○	○	○	○	○	○	○
W	○	○	○	○	○	○	○
T	○	○	○	○	○	○	○
F	○	○	○	○	○	○	○
S a	○	○	○	○	○	○	○
S u	○	○	○	○	○	○	○

SHOPPING LIST

-
-
-
-
-
-
-
-
-
-

DATE	MONDAY
B'Fast	
Lunch	
Dinner	
Snacks	

DATE	TUESDAY
B'Fast	
Lunch	
Dinner	
Snacks	

DATE	WEDNESDAY
B'Fast	
Lunch	
Dinner	
Snacks	

DATE	THURSDAY
B'Fast	
Lunch	
Dinner	
Snacks	

WEEK	DATE	WEIGHT	+/-

HEALTH GOALS

	FRIDAY	DATE
B'Fast		
Lunch		
Dinner		
Snacks		

	SATURDAY	DATE
B'Fast		
Lunch		
Dinner		
Snacks		

	SUNDAY	DATE
B'Fast		
Lunch		
Dinner		
Snacks		

WATER TRACKER

M	○	○	○	○	○	○	○
T	○	○	○	○	○	○	○
W	○	○	○	○	○	○	○
T	○	○	○	○	○	○	○
F	○	○	○	○	○	○	○
Sa	○	○	○	○	○	○	○
Su	○	○	○	○	○	○	○

SHOPPING LIST

-
-
-
-
-
-
-
-
-

DATE	MONDAY
B'Fast	
Lunch	
Dinner	
Snacks	

DATE	TUESDAY
B'Fast	
Lunch	
Dinner	
Snacks	

DATE	WEDNESDAY
B'Fast	
Lunch	
Dinner	
Snacks	

DATE	THURSDAY
B'Fast	
Lunch	
Dinner	
Snacks	

WEEK	DATE	WEIGHT	+/-

HEALTH GOALS

FRIDAY		DATE
B'Fast		
Lunch		
Dinner		
Snacks		

SATURDAY		DATE
B'Fast		
Lunch		
Dinner		
Snacks		

SUNDAY		DATE
B'Fast		
Lunch		
Dinner		
Snacks		

WATER TRACKER

M	○	○	○	○	○	○	○
T	○	○	○	○	○	○	○
W	○	○	○	○	○	○	○
T	○	○	○	○	○	○	○
F	○	○	○	○	○	○	○
Sa	○	○	○	○	○	○	○
Su	○	○	○	○	○	○	○

SHOPPING LIST

-
-
-
-
-
-
-
-
-
-

DATE	MONDAY
B'Fast	
Lunch	
Dinner	
Snacks	

DATE	TUESDAY
B'Fast	
Lunch	
Dinner	
Snacks	

DATE	WEDNESDAY
B'Fast	
Lunch	
Dinner	
Snacks	

DATE	THURSDAY
B'Fast	
Lunch	
Dinner	
Snacks	

WEEK	DATE	WEIGHT	+/-

HEALTH GOALS

	FRIDAY	DATE
B'Fast		
Lunch		
Dinner		
Snacks		

	SATURDAY	DATE
B'Fast		
Lunch		
Dinner		
Snacks		

	SUNDAY	DATE
B'Fast		
Lunch		
Dinner		
Snacks		

WATER TRACKER

M	○	○	○	○	○	○	○
T	○	○	○	○	○	○	○
W	○	○	○	○	○	○	○
T	○	○	○	○	○	○	○
F	○	○	○	○	○	○	○
Sa	○	○	○	○	○	○	○
Su	○	○	○	○	○	○	○

SHOPPING LIST

-
-
-
-
-
-
-
-
-

DATE	MONDAY
B'Fast	
Lunch	
Dinner	
Snacks	

DATE	TUESDAY
B'Fast	
Lunch	
Dinner	
Snacks	

DATE	WEDNESDAY
B'Fast	
Lunch	
Dinner	
Snacks	

DATE	THURSDAY
B'Fast	
Lunch	
Dinner	
Snacks	

WEEK	DATE	WEIGHT	+/-

HEALTH GOALS

	FRIDAY	DATE
B'Fast		
Lunch		
Dinner		
Snacks		

	SATURDAY	DATE
B'Fast		
Lunch		
Dinner		
Snacks		

	SUNDAY	DATE
B'Fast		
Lunch		
Dinner		
Snacks		

WATER TRACKER

M	○	○	○	○	○	○	○
T	○	○	○	○	○	○	○
W	○	○	○	○	○	○	○
T	○	○	○	○	○	○	○
F	○	○	○	○	○	○	○
Sa	○	○	○	○	○	○	○
Su	○	○	○	○	○	○	○

SHOPPING LIST

-
-
-
-
-
-
-
-
-
-

DATE	MONDAY
B'Fast	
Lunch	
Dinner	
Snacks	

DATE	TUESDAY
B'Fast	
Lunch	
Dinner	
Snacks	

DATE	WEDNESDAY
B'Fast	
Lunch	
Dinner	
Snacks	

DATE	THURSDAY
B'Fast	
Lunch	
Dinner	
Snacks	

WEEK	DATE	WEIGHT	+/-

HEALTH GOALS

	FRIDAY	**DATE**
B'Fast		
Lunch		
Dinner		
Snacks		

	SATURDAY	**DATE**
B'Fast		
Lunch		
Dinner		
Snacks		

	SUNDAY	**DATE**
B'Fast		
Lunch		
Dinner		
Snacks		

WATER TRACKER

M	○	○	○	○	○	○	○
T	○	○	○	○	○	○	○
W	○	○	○	○	○	○	○
T	○	○	○	○	○	○	○
F	○	○	○	○	○	○	○
Sa	○	○	○	○	○	○	○
Su	○	○	○	○	○	○	○

SHOPPING LIST

-
-
-
-
-
-
-
-
-
-

DATE	MONDAY
B'Fast	
Lunch	
Dinner	
Snacks	

DATE	TUESDAY
B'Fast	
Lunch	
Dinner	
Snacks	

DATE	WEDNESDAY
B'Fast	
Lunch	
Dinner	
Snacks	

DATE	THURSDAY
B'Fast	
Lunch	
Dinner	
Snacks	

WEEK	DATE	WEIGHT	+/-

HEALTH GOALS

	FRIDAY	DATE
B'Fast		
Lunch		
Dinner		
Snacks		

	SATURDAY	DATE
B'Fast		
Lunch		
Dinner		
Snacks		

	SUNDAY	DATE
B'Fast		
Lunch		
Dinner		
Snacks		

WATER TRACKER

M	○	○	○	○	○	○	○
T	○	○	○	○	○	○	○
W	○	○	○	○	○	○	○
T	○	○	○	○	○	○	○
F	○	○	○	○	○	○	○
S a	○	○	○	○	○	○	○
S u	○	○	○	○	○	○	○

SHOPPING LIST

-
-
-
-
-
-
-
-
-
-

DATE	MONDAY
B'Fast	
Lunch	
Dinner	
Snacks	

DATE	TUESDAY
B'Fast	
Lunch	
Dinner	
Snacks	

DATE	WEDNESDAY
B'Fast	
Lunch	
Dinner	
Snacks	

DATE	THURSDAY
B'Fast	
Lunch	
Dinner	
Snacks	

WEEK	DATE	WEIGHT	+/-

HEALTH GOALS

FRIDAY	DATE
B'Fast	
Lunch	
Dinner	
Snacks	

SATURDAY	DATE
B'Fast	
Lunch	
Dinner	
Snacks	

SUNDAY	DATE
B'Fast	
Lunch	
Dinner	
Snacks	

WATER TRACKER

M	○	○	○	○	○	○	○
T	○	○	○	○	○	○	○
W	○	○	○	○	○	○	○
T	○	○	○	○	○	○	○
F	○	○	○	○	○	○	○
Sa	○	○	○	○	○	○	○
Su	○	○	○	○	○	○	○

SHOPPING LIST

-
-
-
-
-
-
-
-
-
-

DATE	MONDAY
B'Fast	
Lunch	
Dinner	
Snacks	

DATE	TUESDAY
B'Fast	
Lunch	
Dinner	
Snacks	

DATE	WEDNESDAY
B'Fast	
Lunch	
Dinner	
Snacks	

DATE	THURSDAY
B'Fast	
Lunch	
Dinner	
Snacks	

WEEK	DATE	WEIGHT	+/-

HEALTH GOALS

FRIDAY	DATE
B'Fast	
Lunch	
Dinner	
Snacks	

SATURDAY	DATE
B'Fast	
Lunch	
Dinner	
Snacks	

SUNDAY	DATE
B'Fast	
Lunch	
Dinner	
Snacks	

WATER TRACKER

M	○	○	○	○	○	○	○
T	○	○	○	○	○	○	○
W	○	○	○	○	○	○	○
T	○	○	○	○	○	○	○
F	○	○	○	○	○	○	○
Sa	○	○	○	○	○	○	○
Su	○	○	○	○	○	○	○

SHOPPING LIST

-
-
-
-
-
-
-
-
-
-

DATE	MONDAY
B'Fast	
Lunch	
Dinner	
Snacks	

DATE	TUESDAY
B'Fast	
Lunch	
Dinner	
Snacks	

DATE	WEDNESDAY
B'Fast	
Lunch	
Dinner	
Snacks	

DATE	THURSDAY
B'Fast	
Lunch	
Dinner	
Snacks	

WEEK	DATE	WEIGHT	+/-

HEALTH GOALS

FRIDAY	DATE
B'Fast	
Lunch	
Dinner	
Snacks	

SATURDAY	DATE
B'Fast	
Lunch	
Dinner	
Snacks	

SUNDAY	DATE
B'Fast	
Lunch	
Dinner	
Snacks	

WATER TRACKER

M	○	○	○	○	○	○	○
T	○	○	○	○	○	○	○
W	○	○	○	○	○	○	○
T	○	○	○	○	○	○	○
F	○	○	○	○	○	○	○
Sa	○	○	○	○	○	○	○
Su	○	○	○	○	○	○	○

SHOPPING LIST

-
-
-
-
-
-
-
-
-
-

DATE		MONDAY
B'Fast		
Lunch		
Dinner		
Snacks		

DATE		TUESDAY
B'Fast		
Lunch		
Dinner		
Snacks		

DATE		WEDNESDAY
B'Fast		
Lunch		
Dinner		
Snacks		

DATE		THURSDAY
B'Fast		
Lunch		
Dinner		
Snacks		

WEEK	DATE	WEIGHT	+/-

HEALTH GOALS

FRIDAY	DATE
B'Fast	
Lunch	
Dinner	
Snacks	

SATURDAY	DATE
B'Fast	
Lunch	
Dinner	
Snacks	

SUNDAY	DATE
B'Fast	
Lunch	
Dinner	
Snacks	

WATER TRACKER

M	○	○	○	○	○	○	○
T	○	○	○	○	○	○	○
W	○	○	○	○	○	○	○
T	○	○	○	○	○	○	○
F	○	○	○	○	○	○	○
Sa	○	○	○	○	○	○	○
Su	○	○	○	○	○	○	○

SHOPPING LIST

-
-
-
-
-
-
-
-
-
-

DATE	MONDAY
B'Fast	
Lunch	
Dinner	
Snacks	

DATE	TUESDAY
B'Fast	
Lunch	
Dinner	
Snacks	

DATE	WEDNESDAY
B'Fast	
Lunch	
Dinner	
Snacks	

DATE	THURSDAY
B'Fast	
Lunch	
Dinner	
Snacks	

WEEK	DATE	WEIGHT	+/-

HEALTH GOALS

	FRIDAY	DATE
B'Fast		
Lunch		
Dinner		
Snacks		

	SATURDAY	DATE
B'Fast		
Lunch		
Dinner		
Snacks		

	SUNDAY	DATE
B'Fast		
Lunch		
Dinner		
Snacks		

WATER TRACKER

M	○	○	○	○	○	○	○
T	○	○	○	○	○	○	○
W	○	○	○	○	○	○	○
T	○	○	○	○	○	○	○
F	○	○	○	○	○	○	○
Sa	○	○	○	○	○	○	○
Su	○	○	○	○	○	○	○

SHOPPING LIST

-
-
-
-
-
-
-
-
-
-

DATE	MONDAY
B'Fast	
Lunch	
Dinner	
Snacks	

DATE	TUESDAY
B'Fast	
Lunch	
Dinner	
Snacks	

DATE	WEDNESDAY
B'Fast	
Lunch	
Dinner	
Snacks	

DATE	THURSDAY
B'Fast	
Lunch	
Dinner	
Snacks	

WEEK	DATE	WEIGHT	+/-

HEALTH GOALS

FRIDAY	DATE
B'Fast	
Lunch	
Dinner	
Snacks	

SATURDAY	DATE
B'Fast	
Lunch	
Dinner	
Snacks	

SUNDAY	DATE
B'Fast	
Lunch	
Dinner	
Snacks	

WATER TRACKER

M	○	○	○	○	○	○	○
T	○	○	○	○	○	○	○
W	○	○	○	○	○	○	○
T	○	○	○	○	○	○	○
F	○	○	○	○	○	○	○
Sa	○	○	○	○	○	○	○
Su	○	○	○	○	○	○	○

SHOPPING LIST

-
-
-
-
-
-
-
-
-
-

DATE	MONDAY		
B'Fast			
Lunch			
Dinner			
Snacks			

DATE	TUESDAY		
B'Fast			
Lunch			
Dinner			
Snacks			

DATE	WEDNESDAY		
B'Fast			
Lunch			
Dinner			
Snacks			

DATE	THURSDAY		
B'Fast			
Lunch			
Dinner			
Snacks			

WEEK	DATE	WEIGHT	+/-

HEALTH GOALS

FRIDAY	DATE
B'Fast	
Lunch	
Dinner	
Snacks	

SATURDAY	DATE
B'Fast	
Lunch	
Dinner	
Snacks	

SUNDAY	DATE
B'Fast	
Lunch	
Dinner	
Snacks	

WATER TRACKER

M	○	○	○	○	○	○	○
T	○	○	○	○	○	○	○
W	○	○	○	○	○	○	○
T	○	○	○	○	○	○	○
F	○	○	○	○	○	○	○
Sa	○	○	○	○	○	○	○
Su	○	○	○	○	○	○	○

SHOPPING LIST

-
-
-
-
-
-
-
-
-
-

DATE	MONDAY		
B'Fast			
Lunch			
Dinner			
Snacks			

DATE	TUESDAY		
B'Fast			
Lunch			
Dinner			
Snacks			

DATE	WEDNESDAY		
B'Fast			
Lunch			
Dinner			
Snacks			

DATE	THURSDAY		
B'Fast			
Lunch			
Dinner			
Snacks			

WEEK	DATE	WEIGHT	+/-

HEALTH GOALS

	FRIDAY	**DATE**
B'Fast		
Lunch		
Dinner		
Snacks		

	SATURDAY	**DATE**
B'Fast		
Lunch		
Dinner		
Snacks		

	SUNDAY	**DATE**
B'Fast		
Lunch		
Dinner		
Snacks		

WATER TRACKER

M	○	○	○	○	○	○	○
T	○	○	○	○	○	○	○
W	○	○	○	○	○	○	○
T	○	○	○	○	○	○	○
F	○	○	○	○	○	○	○
Sa	○	○	○	○	○	○	○
Su	○	○	○	○	○	○	○

SHOPPING LIST

-
-
-
-
-
-
-
-
-

DATE	MONDAY
B'Fast	
Lunch	
Dinner	
Snacks	

DATE	TUESDAY
B'Fast	
Lunch	
Dinner	
Snacks	

DATE	WEDNESDAY
B'Fast	
Lunch	
Dinner	
Snacks	

DATE	THURSDAY
B'Fast	
Lunch	
Dinner	
Snacks	

WEEK	DATE	WEIGHT	+/-

HEALTH GOALS

	FRIDAY	DATE
B'Fast		
Lunch		
Dinner		
Snacks		

	SATURDAY	DATE
B'Fast		
Lunch		
Dinner		
Snacks		

	SUNDAY	DATE
B'Fast		
Lunch		
Dinner		
Snacks		

WATER TRACKER

M	○	○	○	○	○	○	○
T	○	○	○	○	○	○	○
W	○	○	○	○	○	○	○
T	○	○	○	○	○	○	○
F	○	○	○	○	○	○	○
Sa	○	○	○	○	○	○	○
Su	○	○	○	○	○	○	○

SHOPPING LIST

-
-
-
-
-
-
-
-
-
-

DATE	MONDAY		
B'Fast			
Lunch			
Dinner			
Snacks			

DATE	TUESDAY		
B'Fast			
Lunch			
Dinner			
Snacks			

DATE	WEDNESDAY		
B'Fast			
Lunch			
Dinner			
Snacks			

DATE	THURSDAY		
B'Fast			
Lunch			
Dinner			
Snacks			

WEEK	DATE	WEIGHT	+/-

HEALTH GOALS

FRIDAY	DATE
B'Fast	
Lunch	
Dinner	
Snacks	

SATURDAY	DATE
B'Fast	
Lunch	
Dinner	
Snacks	

SUNDAY	DATE
B'Fast	
Lunch	
Dinner	
Snacks	

WATER TRACKER

M	○	○	○	○	○	○	○
T	○	○	○	○	○	○	○
W	○	○	○	○	○	○	○
T	○	○	○	○	○	○	○
F	○	○	○	○	○	○	○
Sa	○	○	○	○	○	○	○
Su	○	○	○	○	○	○	○

SHOPPING LIST

-
-
-
-
-
-
-
-
-
-

DATE	MONDAY
B'Fast	
Lunch	
Dinner	
Snacks	

DATE	TUESDAY
B'Fast	
Lunch	
Dinner	
Snacks	

DATE	WEDNESDAY
B'Fast	
Lunch	
Dinner	
Snacks	

DATE	THURSDAY
B'Fast	
Lunch	
Dinner	
Snacks	

WEEK	DATE	WEIGHT	+/-

HEALTH GOALS

FRIDAY	DATE
B'Fast	
Lunch	
Dinner	
Snacks	

SATURDAY	DATE
B'Fast	
Lunch	
Dinner	
Snacks	

SUNDAY	DATE
B'Fast	
Lunch	
Dinner	
Snacks	

WATER TRACKER

M	○	○	○	○	○	○	○
T	○	○	○	○	○	○	○
W	○	○	○	○	○	○	○
T	○	○	○	○	○	○	○
F	○	○	○	○	○	○	○
Sa	○	○	○	○	○	○	○
Su	○	○	○	○	○	○	○

SHOPPING LIST

-
-
-
-
-
-
-
-
-

DATE	MONDAY
B'Fast	
Lunch	
Dinner	
Snacks	

DATE	TUESDAY
B'Fast	
Lunch	
Dinner	
Snacks	

DATE	WEDNESDAY
B'Fast	
Lunch	
Dinner	
Snacks	

DATE	THURSDAY
B'Fast	
Lunch	
Dinner	
Snacks	

WEEK	DATE	WEIGHT	+/-

HEALTH GOALS

	FRIDAY	DATE
B'Fast		
Lunch		
Dinner		
Snacks		

	SATURDAY	DATE
B'Fast		
Lunch		
Dinner		
Snacks		

	SUNDAY	DATE
B'Fast		
Lunch		
Dinner		
Snacks		

WATER TRACKER

M	○	○	○	○	○	○	○
T	○	○	○	○	○	○	○
W	○	○	○	○	○	○	○
T	○	○	○	○	○	○	○
F	○	○	○	○	○	○	○
Sa	○	○	○	○	○	○	○
Su	○	○	○	○	○	○	○

SHOPPING LIST

-
-
-
-
-
-
-
-
-
-

DATE	MONDAY		
B'Fast			
Lunch			
Dinner			
Snacks			

DATE	TUESDAY		
B'Fast			
Lunch			
Dinner			
Snacks			

DATE	WEDNESDAY		
B'Fast			
Lunch			
Dinner			
Snacks			

DATE	THURSDAY		
B'Fast			
Lunch			
Dinner			
Snacks			

WEEK	DATE	WEIGHT	+/-

HEALTH GOALS

	FRIDAY	DATE
B'Fast		
Lunch		
Dinner		
Snacks		

	SATURDAY	DATE
B'Fast		
Lunch		
Dinner		
Snacks		

	SUNDAY	DATE
B'Fast		
Lunch		
Dinner		
Snacks		

WATER TRACKER

M	○	○	○	○	○	○	○
T	○	○	○	○	○	○	○
W	○	○	○	○	○	○	○
T	○	○	○	○	○	○	○
F	○	○	○	○	○	○	○
Sa	○	○	○	○	○	○	○
Su	○	○	○	○	○	○	○

SHOPPING LIST

-
-
-
-
-
-
-
-
-
-

DATE	MONDAY		
B'Fast			
Lunch			
Dinner			
Snacks			

DATE	TUESDAY		
B'Fast			
Lunch			
Dinner			
Snacks			

DATE	WEDNESDAY		
B'Fast			
Lunch			
Dinner			
Snacks			

DATE	THURSDAY		
B'Fast			
Lunch			
Dinner			
Snacks			

WEEK	DATE	WEIGHT	+/-

HEALTH GOALS

FRIDAY		DATE	
B'Fast			
Lunch			
Dinner			
Snacks			

SATURDAY		DATE	
B'Fast			
Lunch			
Dinner			
Snacks			

SUNDAY		DATE	
B'Fast			
Lunch			
Dinner			
Snacks			

WATER TRACKER

M	○	○	○	○	○	○	○
T	○	○	○	○	○	○	○
W	○	○	○	○	○	○	○
T	○	○	○	○	○	○	○
F	○	○	○	○	○	○	○
Sa	○	○	○	○	○	○	○
Su	○	○	○	○	○	○	○

SHOPPING LIST

-
-
-
-
-
-
-
-
-
-

DATE	MONDAY
B'Fast	
Lunch	
Dinner	
Snacks	

DATE	TUESDAY
B'Fast	
Lunch	
Dinner	
Snacks	

DATE	WEDNESDAY
B'Fast	
Lunch	
Dinner	
Snacks	

DATE	THURSDAY
B'Fast	
Lunch	
Dinner	
Snacks	

WEEK	DATE	WEIGHT	+/-

HEALTH GOALS

FRIDAY	DATE
B'Fast	
Lunch	
Dinner	
Snacks	

SATURDAY	DATE
B'Fast	
Lunch	
Dinner	
Snacks	

SUNDAY	DATE
B'Fast	
Lunch	
Dinner	
Snacks	

WATER TRACKER

M	○	○	○	○	○	○	○
T	○	○	○	○	○	○	○
W	○	○	○	○	○	○	○
T	○	○	○	○	○	○	○
F	○	○	○	○	○	○	○
Sa	○	○	○	○	○	○	○
Su	○	○	○	○	○	○	○

SHOPPING LIST

-
-
-
-
-
-
-
-
-
-

DATE	MONDAY
B'Fast	
Lunch	
Dinner	
Snacks	

DATE	TUESDAY
B'Fast	
Lunch	
Dinner	
Snacks	

DATE	WEDNESDAY
B'Fast	
Lunch	
Dinner	
Snacks	

DATE	THURSDAY
B'Fast	
Lunch	
Dinner	
Snacks	

WEEK	DATE	WEIGHT	+/-

HEALTH GOALS

	FRIDAY	DATE
B'Fast		
Lunch		
Dinner		
Snacks		

	SATURDAY	DATE
B'Fast		
Lunch		
Dinner		
Snacks		

	SUNDAY	DATE
B'Fast		
Lunch		
Dinner		
Snacks		

WATER TRACKER

M	○	○	○	○	○	○	○
T	○	○	○	○	○	○	○
W	○	○	○	○	○	○	○
T	○	○	○	○	○	○	○
F	○	○	○	○	○	○	○
Sa	○	○	○	○	○	○	○
Su	○	○	○	○	○	○	○

SHOPPING LIST

-
-
-
-
-
-
-
-
-
-

DATE	MONDAY
B'Fast	
Lunch	
Dinner	
Snacks	

DATE	TUESDAY
B'Fast	
Lunch	
Dinner	
Snacks	

DATE	WEDNESDAY
B'Fast	
Lunch	
Dinner	
Snacks	

DATE	THURSDAY
B'Fast	
Lunch	
Dinner	
Snacks	

WEEK	DATE	WEIGHT	+/-

HEALTH GOALS

FRIDAY	DATE
B'Fast	
Lunch	
Dinner	
Snacks	

SATURDAY	DATE
B'Fast	
Lunch	
Dinner	
Snacks	

SUNDAY	DATE
B'Fast	
Lunch	
Dinner	
Snacks	

WATER TRACKER

M	○	○	○	○	○	○	○
T	○	○	○	○	○	○	○
W	○	○	○	○	○	○	○
T	○	○	○	○	○	○	○
F	○	○	○	○	○	○	○
Sa	○	○	○	○	○	○	○
Su	○	○	○	○	○	○	○

SHOPPING LIST

-
-
-
-
-
-
-
-
-
-

DATE	MONDAY
B'Fast	
Lunch	
Dinner	
Snacks	

DATE	TUESDAY
B'Fast	
Lunch	
Dinner	
Snacks	

DATE	WEDNESDAY
B'Fast	
Lunch	
Dinner	
Snacks	

DATE	THURSDAY
B'Fast	
Lunch	
Dinner	
Snacks	

WEEK	DATE	WEIGHT	+/-

HEALTH GOALS

FRIDAY		DATE
B'Fast		
Lunch		
Dinner		
Snacks		

SATURDAY		DATE
B'Fast		
Lunch		
Dinner		
Snacks		

SUNDAY		DATE
B'Fast		
Lunch		
Dinner		
Snacks		

WATER TRACKER

M	○	○	○	○	○	○	○
T	○	○	○	○	○	○	○
W	○	○	○	○	○	○	○
T	○	○	○	○	○	○	○
F	○	○	○	○	○	○	○
Sa	○	○	○	○	○	○	○
Su	○	○	○	○	○	○	○

SHOPPING LIST

-
-
-
-
-
-
-
-
-
-

DATE	MONDAY
B'Fast	
Lunch	
Dinner	
Snacks	

DATE	TUESDAY
B'Fast	
Lunch	
Dinner	
Snacks	

DATE	WEDNESDAY
B'Fast	
Lunch	
Dinner	
Snacks	

DATE	THURSDAY
B'Fast	
Lunch	
Dinner	
Snacks	

WEEK	DATE	WEIGHT	+/-

HEALTH GOALS

	FRIDAY	DATE
B'Fast		
Lunch		
Dinner		
Snacks		

	SATURDAY	DATE
B'Fast		
Lunch		
Dinner		
Snacks		

	SUNDAY	DATE
B'Fast		
Lunch		
Dinner		
Snacks		

WATER TRACKER

M	○	○	○	○	○	○	○
T	○	○	○	○	○	○	○
W	○	○	○	○	○	○	○
T	○	○	○	○	○	○	○
F	○	○	○	○	○	○	○
Sa	○	○	○	○	○	○	○
Su	○	○	○	○	○	○	○

SHOPPING LIST

-
-
-
-
-
-
-
-
-
-

DATE	MONDAY		
B'Fast			
Lunch			
Dinner			
Snacks			

DATE	TUESDAY		
B'Fast			
Lunch			
Dinner			
Snacks			

DATE	WEDNESDAY		
B'Fast			
Lunch			
Dinner			
Snacks			

DATE	THURSDAY		
B'Fast			
Lunch			
Dinner			
Snacks			

WEEK	DATE	WEIGHT	+/-

HEALTH GOALS

FRIDAY	DATE
B'Fast	
Lunch	
Dinner	
Snacks	

SATURDAY	DATE
B'Fast	
Lunch	
Dinner	
Snacks	

SUNDAY	DATE
B'Fast	
Lunch	
Dinner	
Snacks	

WATER TRACKER

M	○	○	○	○	○	○	○
T	○	○	○	○	○	○	○
W	○	○	○	○	○	○	○
T	○	○	○	○	○	○	○
F	○	○	○	○	○	○	○
Sa	○	○	○	○	○	○	○
Su	○	○	○	○	○	○	○

SHOPPING LIST

-
-
-
-
-
-
-
-
-
-

DATE	MONDAY
B'Fast	
Lunch	
Dinner	
Snacks	

DATE	TUESDAY
B'Fast	
Lunch	
Dinner	
Snacks	

DATE	WEDNESDAY
B'Fast	
Lunch	
Dinner	
Snacks	

DATE	THURSDAY
B'Fast	
Lunch	
Dinner	
Snacks	

WEEK	DATE	WEIGHT	+/-

HEALTH GOALS

FRIDAY	**DATE**
B'Fast	
Lunch	
Dinner	
Snacks	

SATURDAY	**DATE**
B'Fast	
Lunch	
Dinner	
Snacks	

SUNDAY	**DATE**
B'Fast	
Lunch	
Dinner	
Snacks	

WATER TRACKER

M	○	○	○	○	○	○	○
T	○	○	○	○	○	○	○
W	○	○	○	○	○	○	○
T	○	○	○	○	○	○	○
F	○	○	○	○	○	○	○
Sa	○	○	○	○	○	○	○
Su	○	○	○	○	○	○	○

SHOPPING LIST

-
-
-
-
-
-
-
-
-
-

DATE	MONDAY
B'Fast	
Lunch	
Dinner	
Snacks	

DATE	TUESDAY
B'Fast	
Lunch	
Dinner	
Snacks	

DATE	WEDNESDAY
B'Fast	
Lunch	
Dinner	
Snacks	

DATE	THURSDAY
B'Fast	
Lunch	
Dinner	
Snacks	

WEEK	DATE	WEIGHT	+/-

HEALTH GOALS

FRIDAY	DATE
B'Fast	
Lunch	
Dinner	
Snacks	

SATURDAY	DATE
B'Fast	
Lunch	
Dinner	
Snacks	

SUNDAY	DATE
B'Fast	
Lunch	
Dinner	
Snacks	

WATER TRACKER

M	○	○	○	○	○	○	○
T	○	○	○	○	○	○	○
W	○	○	○	○	○	○	○
T	○	○	○	○	○	○	○
F	○	○	○	○	○	○	○
Sa	○	○	○	○	○	○	○
Su	○	○	○	○	○	○	○

SHOPPING LIST

-
-
-
-
-
-
-
-
-
-

DATE	MONDAY
B'Fast	
Lunch	
Dinner	
Snacks	

DATE	TUESDAY
B'Fast	
Lunch	
Dinner	
Snacks	

DATE	WEDNESDAY
B'Fast	
Lunch	
Dinner	
Snacks	

DATE	THURSDAY
B'Fast	
Lunch	
Dinner	
Snacks	

WEEK	DATE	WEIGHT	+/-

HEALTH GOALS

FRIDAY	DATE
B'Fast	
Lunch	
Dinner	
Snacks	

SATURDAY	DATE
B'Fast	
Lunch	
Dinner	
Snacks	

SUNDAY	DATE
B'Fast	
Lunch	
Dinner	
Snacks	

WATER TRACKER

M	○	○	○	○	○	○	○
T	○	○	○	○	○	○	○
W	○	○	○	○	○	○	○
T	○	○	○	○	○	○	○
F	○	○	○	○	○	○	○
Sa	○	○	○	○	○	○	○
Su	○	○	○	○	○	○	○

SHOPPING LIST

-
-
-
-
-
-
-
-
-
-

DATE	MONDAY
B'Fast	
Lunch	
Dinner	
Snacks	

DATE	TUESDAY
B'Fast	
Lunch	
Dinner	
Snacks	

DATE	WEDNESDAY
B'Fast	
Lunch	
Dinner	
Snacks	

DATE	THURSDAY
B'Fast	
Lunch	
Dinner	
Snacks	

WEEK	DATE	WEIGHT	+/-

HEALTH GOALS

FRIDAY	DATE
B'Fast	
Lunch	
Dinner	
Snacks	

SATURDAY	DATE
B'Fast	
Lunch	
Dinner	
Snacks	

SUNDAY	DATE
B'Fast	
Lunch	
Dinner	
Snacks	

WATER TRACKER

M	○	○	○	○	○	○	○
T	○	○	○	○	○	○	○
W	○	○	○	○	○	○	○
T	○	○	○	○	○	○	○
F	○	○	○	○	○	○	○
Sa	○	○	○	○	○	○	○
Su	○	○	○	○	○	○	○

SHOPPING LIST

-
-
-
-
-
-
-
-
-
-

DATE	MONDAY		
B'Fast			
Lunch			
Dinner			
Snacks			

DATE	TUESDAY		
B'Fast			
Lunch			
Dinner			
Snacks			

DATE	WEDNESDAY		
B'Fast			
Lunch			
Dinner			
Snacks			

DATE	THURSDAY		
B'Fast			
Lunch			
Dinner			
Snacks			

WEEK	DATE	WEIGHT	+/-

HEALTH GOALS

	FRIDAY	DATE
B'Fast		
Lunch		
Dinner		
Snacks		

	SATURDAY	DATE
B'Fast		
Lunch		
Dinner		
Snacks		

	SUNDAY	DATE
B'Fast		
Lunch		
Dinner		
Snacks		

WATER TRACKER

M	○	○	○	○	○	○	○
T	○	○	○	○	○	○	○
W	○	○	○	○	○	○	○
T	○	○	○	○	○	○	○
F	○	○	○	○	○	○	○
Sa	○	○	○	○	○	○	○
Su	○	○	○	○	○	○	○

SHOPPING LIST

-
-
-
-
-
-
-
-
-
-

DATE	MONDAY
B'Fast	
Lunch	
Dinner	
Snacks	

DATE	TUESDAY
B'Fast	
Lunch	
Dinner	
Snacks	

DATE	WEDNESDAY
B'Fast	
Lunch	
Dinner	
Snacks	

DATE	THURSDAY
B'Fast	
Lunch	
Dinner	
Snacks	

WEEK	DATE	WEIGHT	+/-

HEALTH GOALS

FRIDAY		DATE
B'Fast		
Lunch		
Dinner		
Snacks		

SATURDAY		DATE
B'Fast		
Lunch		
Dinner		
Snacks		

SUNDAY		DATE
B'Fast		
Lunch		
Dinner		
Snacks		

WATER TRACKER

M	○	○	○	○	○	○	○
T	○	○	○	○	○	○	○
W	○	○	○	○	○	○	○
T	○	○	○	○	○	○	○
F	○	○	○	○	○	○	○
Sa	○	○	○	○	○	○	○
Su	○	○	○	○	○	○	○

SHOPPING LIST

-
-
-
-
-
-
-
-
-
-

DATE	**MONDAY**
B'Fast	
Lunch	
Dinner	
Snacks	

DATE	**TUESDAY**
B'Fast	
Lunch	
Dinner	
Snacks	

DATE	**WEDNESDAY**
B'Fast	
Lunch	
Dinner	
Snacks	

DATE	**THURSDAY**
B'Fast	
Lunch	
Dinner	
Snacks	

WEEK	DATE	WEIGHT	+/-

<u>HEALTH GOALS</u>

FRIDAY	DATE
B'Fast	
Lunch	
Dinner	
Snacks	

SATURDAY	DATE
B'Fast	
Lunch	
Dinner	
Snacks	

SUNDAY	DATE
B'Fast	
Lunch	
Dinner	
Snacks	

WATER TRACKER

M	○	○	○	○	○	○	○
T	○	○	○	○	○	○	○
W	○	○	○	○	○	○	○
T	○	○	○	○	○	○	○
F	○	○	○	○	○	○	○
Sa	○	○	○	○	○	○	○
Su	○	○	○	○	○	○	○

SHOPPING LIST

-
-
-
-
-
-
-
-
-
-

DATE	MONDAY
B'Fast	
Lunch	
Dinner	
Snacks	

DATE	TUESDAY
B'Fast	
Lunch	
Dinner	
Snacks	

DATE	WEDNESDAY
B'Fast	
Lunch	
Dinner	
Snacks	

DATE	THURSDAY
B'Fast	
Lunch	
Dinner	
Snacks	

WEEK	DATE	WEIGHT	+/-

HEALTH GOALS

	FRIDAY	DATE
B'Fast		
Lunch		
Dinner		
Snacks		

	SATURDAY	DATE
B'Fast		
Lunch		
Dinner		
Snacks		

	SUNDAY	DATE
B'Fast		
Lunch		
Dinner		
Snacks		

WATER TRACKER

M	○	○	○	○	○	○	○
T	○	○	○	○	○	○	○
W	○	○	○	○	○	○	○
T	○	○	○	○	○	○	○
F	○	○	○	○	○	○	○
S a	○	○	○	○	○	○	○
S u	○	○	○	○	○	○	○

SHOPPING LIST

-
-
-
-
-
-
-
-
-
-

DATE	MONDAY
B'Fast	
Lunch	
Dinner	
Snacks	

DATE	TUESDAY
B'Fast	
Lunch	
Dinner	
Snacks	

DATE	WEDNESDAY
B'Fast	
Lunch	
Dinner	
Snacks	

DATE	THURSDAY
B'Fast	
Lunch	
Dinner	
Snacks	

WEEK	DATE	WEIGHT	+/-

HEALTH GOALS

FRIDAY	DATE
B'Fast	
Lunch	
Dinner	
Snacks	

SATURDAY	DATE
B'Fast	
Lunch	
Dinner	
Snacks	

SUNDAY	DATE
B'Fast	
Lunch	
Dinner	
Snacks	

WATER TRACKER

M	○	○	○	○	○	○	○
T	○	○	○	○	○	○	○
W	○	○	○	○	○	○	○
T	○	○	○	○	○	○	○
F	○	○	○	○	○	○	○
Sa	○	○	○	○	○	○	○
Su	○	○	○	○	○	○	○

SHOPPING LIST

-
-
-
-
-
-
-
-
-
-

DATE	MONDAY
B'Fast	
Lunch	
Dinner	
Snacks	

DATE	TUESDAY
B'Fast	
Lunch	
Dinner	
Snacks	

DATE	WEDNESDAY
B'Fast	
Lunch	
Dinner	
Snacks	

DATE	THURSDAY
B'Fast	
Lunch	
Dinner	
Snacks	

WEEK	DATE	WEIGHT	+/-

HEALTH GOALS

FRIDAY	DATE
B'Fast	
Lunch	
Dinner	
Snacks	

SATURDAY	DATE
B'Fast	
Lunch	
Dinner	
Snacks	

SUNDAY	DATE
B'Fast	
Lunch	
Dinner	
Snacks	

WATER TRACKER

M	○	○	○	○	○	○	○
T	○	○	○	○	○	○	○
W	○	○	○	○	○	○	○
T	○	○	○	○	○	○	○
F	○	○	○	○	○	○	○
Sa	○	○	○	○	○	○	○
Su	○	○	○	○	○	○	○

SHOPPING LIST

-
-
-
-
-
-
-
-
-
-

DATE	MONDAY
B'Fast	
Lunch	
Dinner	
Snacks	

DATE	TUESDAY
B'Fast	
Lunch	
Dinner	
Snacks	

DATE	WEDNESDAY
B'Fast	
Lunch	
Dinner	
Snacks	

DATE	THURSDAY
B'Fast	
Lunch	
Dinner	
Snacks	

WEEK	DATE	WEIGHT	+/-

HEALTH GOALS

FRIDAY	DATE
B'Fast	
Lunch	
Dinner	
Snacks	

SATURDAY	DATE
B'Fast	
Lunch	
Dinner	
Snacks	

SUNDAY	DATE
B'Fast	
Lunch	
Dinner	
Snacks	

WATER TRACKER

M	○	○	○	○	○	○	○
T	○	○	○	○	○	○	○
W	○	○	○	○	○	○	○
T	○	○	○	○	○	○	○
F	○	○	○	○	○	○	○
Sa	○	○	○	○	○	○	○
Su	○	○	○	○	○	○	○

SHOPPING LIST

-
-
-
-
-
-
-
-
-
-

DATE	MONDAY
B'Fast	
Lunch	
Dinner	
Snacks	

DATE	TUESDAY
B'Fast	
Lunch	
Dinner	
Snacks	

DATE	WEDNESDAY
B'Fast	
Lunch	
Dinner	
Snacks	

DATE	THURSDAY
B'Fast	
Lunch	
Dinner	
Snacks	

WEEK	DATE	WEIGHT	+/-

HEALTH GOALS

FRIDAY	DATE
B'Fast	
Lunch	
Dinner	
Snacks	

SATURDAY	DATE
B'Fast	
Lunch	
Dinner	
Snacks	

SUNDAY	DATE
B'Fast	
Lunch	
Dinner	
Snacks	

WATER TRACKER

M	○	○	○	○	○	○	○
T	○	○	○	○	○	○	○
W	○	○	○	○	○	○	○
T	○	○	○	○	○	○	○
F	○	○	○	○	○	○	○
Sa	○	○	○	○	○	○	○
Su	○	○	○	○	○	○	○

SHOPPING LIST

-
-
-
-
-
-
-
-
-
-

DATE	MONDAY
B'Fast	
Lunch	
Dinner	
Snacks	

DATE	TUESDAY
B'Fast	
Lunch	
Dinner	
Snacks	

DATE	WEDNESDAY
B'Fast	
Lunch	
Dinner	
Snacks	

DATE	THURSDAY
B'Fast	
Lunch	
Dinner	
Snacks	

WEEK	DATE	WEIGHT	+/-

HEALTH GOALS

	FRIDAY	DATE
B'Fast		
Lunch		
Dinner		
Snacks		

	SATURDAY	DATE
B'Fast		
Lunch		
Dinner		
Snacks		

	SUNDAY	DATE
B'Fast		
Lunch		
Dinner		
Snacks		

WATER TRACKER

M	○	○	○	○	○	○	○
T	○	○	○	○	○	○	○
W	○	○	○	○	○	○	○
T	○	○	○	○	○	○	○
F	○	○	○	○	○	○	○
S a	○	○	○	○	○	○	○
S u	○	○	○	○	○	○	○

SHOPPING LIST

-
-
-
-
-
-
-
-
-
-

DATE	MONDAY
B'Fast	
Lunch	
Dinner	
Snacks	

DATE	TUESDAY
B'Fast	
Lunch	
Dinner	
Snacks	

DATE	WEDNESDAY
B'Fast	
Lunch	
Dinner	
Snacks	

DATE	THURSDAY
B'Fast	
Lunch	
Dinner	
Snacks	

WEEK	DATE	WEIGHT	+/-

HEALTH GOALS

FRIDAY		DATE
B'Fast		
Lunch		
Dinner		
Snacks		

SATURDAY		DATE
B'Fast		
Lunch		
Dinner		
Snacks		

SUNDAY		DATE
B'Fast		
Lunch		
Dinner		
Snacks		

WATER TRACKER

M	○	○	○	○	○	○	○
T	○	○	○	○	○	○	○
W	○	○	○	○	○	○	○
T	○	○	○	○	○	○	○
F	○	○	○	○	○	○	○
Sa	○	○	○	○	○	○	○
Su	○	○	○	○	○	○	○

SHOPPING LIST

-
-
-
-
-
-
-
-
-
-

DATE	MONDAY
B'Fast	
Lunch	
Dinner	
Snacks	

DATE	TUESDAY
B'Fast	
Lunch	
Dinner	
Snacks	

DATE	WEDNESDAY
B'Fast	
Lunch	
Dinner	
Snacks	

DATE	THURSDAY
B'Fast	
Lunch	
Dinner	
Snacks	

WEEK	DATE	WEIGHT	+/-

HEALTH GOALS

FRIDAY		DATE
B'Fast		
Lunch		
Dinner		
Snacks		

SATURDAY		DATE
B'Fast		
Lunch		
Dinner		
Snacks		

SUNDAY		DATE
B'Fast		
Lunch		
Dinner		
Snacks		

WATER TRACKER

M	○	○	○	○	○	○	○
T	○	○	○	○	○	○	○
W	○	○	○	○	○	○	○
T	○	○	○	○	○	○	○
F	○	○	○	○	○	○	○
Sa	○	○	○	○	○	○	○
Su	○	○	○	○	○	○	○

SHOPPING LIST

-
-
-
-
-
-
-
-
-
-

DATE	MONDAY		
B'Fast			
Lunch			
Dinner			
Snacks			

DATE	TUESDAY		
B'Fast			
Lunch			
Dinner			
Snacks			

DATE	WEDNESDAY		
B'Fast			
Lunch			
Dinner			
Snacks			

DATE	THURSDAY		
B'Fast			
Lunch			
Dinner			
Snacks			

WEEK	DATE	WEIGHT	+/-

HEALTH GOALS

	FRIDAY	DATE
B'Fast		
Lunch		
Dinner		
Snacks		

	SATURDAY	DATE
B'Fast		
Lunch		
Dinner		
Snacks		

	SUNDAY	DATE
B'Fast		
Lunch		
Dinner		
Snacks		

WATER TRACKER

M	○	○	○	○	○	○	○
T	○	○	○	○	○	○	○
W	○	○	○	○	○	○	○
T	○	○	○	○	○	○	○
F	○	○	○	○	○	○	○
Sa	○	○	○	○	○	○	○
Su	○	○	○	○	○	○	○

SHOPPING LIST

-
-
-
-
-
-
-
-
-
-

DATE	MONDAY
B'Fast	
Lunch	
Dinner	
Snacks	

DATE	TUESDAY
B'Fast	
Lunch	
Dinner	
Snacks	

DATE	WEDNESDAY
B'Fast	
Lunch	
Dinner	
Snacks	

DATE	THURSDAY
B'Fast	
Lunch	
Dinner	
Snacks	

WEEK	DATE	WEIGHT	+/-

HEALTH GOALS

	FRIDAY	DATE
B'Fast		
Lunch		
Dinner		
Snacks		

	SATURDAY	DATE
B'Fast		
Lunch		
Dinner		
Snacks		

	SUNDAY	DATE
B'Fast		
Lunch		
Dinner		
Snacks		

WATER TRACKER

M	○	○	○	○	○	○	○
T	○	○	○	○	○	○	○
W	○	○	○	○	○	○	○
T	○	○	○	○	○	○	○
F	○	○	○	○	○	○	○
Sa	○	○	○	○	○	○	○
Su	○	○	○	○	○	○	○

SHOPPING LIST

-
-
-
-
-
-
-
-
-
-

DATE	MONDAY
B'Fast	
Lunch	
Dinner	
Snacks	

DATE	TUESDAY
B'Fast	
Lunch	
Dinner	
Snacks	

DATE	WEDNESDAY
B'Fast	
Lunch	
Dinner	
Snacks	

DATE	THURSDAY
B'Fast	
Lunch	
Dinner	
Snacks	

WEEK	DATE	WEIGHT	+/-

HEALTH GOALS

FRIDAY	DATE
B'Fast	
Lunch	
Dinner	
Snacks	

SATURDAY	DATE
B'Fast	
Lunch	
Dinner	
Snacks	

SUNDAY	DATE
B'Fast	
Lunch	
Dinner	
Snacks	

WATER TRACKER

M	○	○	○	○	○	○	○
T	○	○	○	○	○	○	○
W	○	○	○	○	○	○	○
T	○	○	○	○	○	○	○
F	○	○	○	○	○	○	○
S a	○	○	○	○	○	○	○
S u	○	○	○	○	○	○	○

SHOPPING LIST

-
-
-
-
-
-
-
-
-
-

DATE	MONDAY
B'Fast	
Lunch	
Dinner	
Snacks	

DATE	TUESDAY
B'Fast	
Lunch	
Dinner	
Snacks	

DATE	WEDNESDAY
B'Fast	
Lunch	
Dinner	
Snacks	

DATE	THURSDAY
B'Fast	
Lunch	
Dinner	
Snacks	

WEEK	DATE	WEIGHT	+/-

HEALTH GOALS

	FRIDAY	DATE
B'Fast		
Lunch		
Dinner		
Snacks		

	SATURDAY	DATE
B'Fast		
Lunch		
Dinner		
Snacks		

	SUNDAY	DATE
B'Fast		
Lunch		
Dinner		
Snacks		

WATER TRACKER

M	○	○	○	○	○	○	○
T	○	○	○	○	○	○	○
W	○	○	○	○	○	○	○
T	○	○	○	○	○	○	○
F	○	○	○	○	○	○	○
Sa	○	○	○	○	○	○	○
Su	○	○	○	○	○	○	○

SHOPPING LIST

-
-
-
-
-
-
-
-
-
-

DATE	MONDAY
B'Fast	
Lunch	
Dinner	
Snacks	

DATE	TUESDAY
B'Fast	
Lunch	
Dinner	
Snacks	

DATE	WEDNESDAY
B'Fast	
Lunch	
Dinner	
Snacks	

DATE	THURSDAY
B'Fast	
Lunch	
Dinner	
Snacks	

WEEK	DATE	WEIGHT	+/-

HEALTH GOALS

	FRIDAY	DATE
B'Fast		
Lunch		
Dinner		
Snacks		

	SATURDAY	DATE
B'Fast		
Lunch		
Dinner		
Snacks		

	SUNDAY	DATE
B'Fast		
Lunch		
Dinner		
Snacks		

WATER TRACKER

M	○	○	○	○	○	○	○
T	○	○	○	○	○	○	○
W	○	○	○	○	○	○	○
T	○	○	○	○	○	○	○
F	○	○	○	○	○	○	○
Sa	○	○	○	○	○	○	○
Su	○	○	○	○	○	○	○

SHOPPING LIST

-
-
-
-
-
-
-
-
-
-

DATE	MONDAY		
B'Fast			
Lunch			
Dinner			
Snacks			

DATE	TUESDAY		
B'Fast			
Lunch			
Dinner			
Snacks			

DATE	WEDNESDAY		
B'Fast			
Lunch			
Dinner			
Snacks			

DATE	THURSDAY		
B'Fast			
Lunch			
Dinner			
Snacks			

WEEK	DATE	WEIGHT	+/-

HEALTH GOALS

FRIDAY	DATE
B'Fast	
Lunch	
Dinner	
Snacks	

SATURDAY	DATE
B'Fast	
Lunch	
Dinner	
Snacks	

SUNDAY	DATE
B'Fast	
Lunch	
Dinner	
Snacks	

WATER TRACKER

M	○	○	○	○	○	○	○
T	○	○	○	○	○	○	○
W	○	○	○	○	○	○	○
T	○	○	○	○	○	○	○
F	○	○	○	○	○	○	○
Sa	○	○	○	○	○	○	○
Su	○	○	○	○	○	○	○

SHOPPING LIST

-
-
-
-
-
-
-
-
-
-

DATE	MONDAY		
B'Fast			
Lunch			
Dinner			
Snacks			

DATE	TUESDAY		
B'Fast			
Lunch			
Dinner			
Snacks			

DATE	WEDNESDAY		
B'Fast			
Lunch			
Dinner			
Snacks			

DATE	THURSDAY		
B'Fast			
Lunch			
Dinner			
Snacks			

WEEK	DATE	WEIGHT	+/-

HEALTH GOALS

	FRIDAY	DATE
B'Fast		
Lunch		
Dinner		
Snacks		

	SATURDAY	DATE
B'Fast		
Lunch		
Dinner		
Snacks		

	SUNDAY	DATE
B'Fast		
Lunch		
Dinner		
Snacks		

WATER TRACKER

M	○	○	○	○	○	○	○
T	○	○	○	○	○	○	○
W	○	○	○	○	○	○	○
T	○	○	○	○	○	○	○
F	○	○	○	○	○	○	○
Sa	○	○	○	○	○	○	○
Su	○	○	○	○	○	○	○

SHOPPING LIST

-
-
-
-
-
-
-
-
-
-

MONTHLY WEIGHT TRACKER

TARGET WEIGHT

MONTH	DATE	WEIGHT	+/-	NOTES
1				
2				
3				
4				
5				
6				
7				
8				
9				
10				
11				
12				

REVIEW / GOALS

Made in the USA
Las Vegas, NV
29 December 2024

15594520R00066